MW00354214

Keep Sharp Recipes:

Easy and Delicious Recipes To Help You Build a Better Brain at Any Age.

By

Roger Press

ISBN: 978-1-954432-14-7

CONTENTS

INTRODUCTION 7

SMART EATING 9

SECRET 1: GO MEDITERRANEAN. 11

SECRET 2: RAMP UP FOODS RICH IN OMEGA-3S. 13

SECRET 2: BINGE ON HEALTHY FRUITS 15

SECRET 4: CUT BACK ON RED MEAT AND DAIRY PRODUCTS. 16

SECRET 5: REDUCE SUGAR AND SIMPLE CARBS. 17

SECRET 6: TAKE THE SALTSHAKER OFF THE TABLE. 19

SECRET 7: SLASH TRANS FATS. 20

CHAPTER 2: KEEP SHARP RECIPES 21

BREAKFAST 21

RECIPES 21

Chick peas and Potato Hash 21

Ingredients: 21

Directions: 22

Avocado Toast 24

INGREDIENTS: 25

DIRECTIONS: 25

MEDITERRANEAN FRITTATA 26

INGREDIENTS: 27

DIRECTIONS: 27

PANCAKES 29

INGREDIENTS: 30

DIRECTIONS: 30

Mediterranean Breakfast Couscous 32

INGREDIENTS: 33

Directions: 33

CHAPTER 3: LUNCH 34

RECIPES: 34

Mango and Black Bean Salad: 34

INGREDIENTS: 35

Chicken, Carrot and Cucumber Salad: 36

INGREDIENTS: 37

DIRECTIONS: 37

Mediterranean Pasta Salad 39

INGREDIENTS: 40

DIRECTIONS: 40

Mediterranean Chickpea Patties 42

INGREDIENTS: 43

DIRECTIONS: 43

Mediterranean shrimp and pasta 45

INGREDIENTS: 46

DIRECTIONS: 46

Mediterranean Pizza 48

INGREDIENTS: 49

DIRECTIONS: 49

CHAPTER 3: DINNER **51**

RECIPES: 51

Mediterranean sea- food grill with skordalia 51

INGREDIENTS: 52

DIRECTIONS: 53

NUTRITIONAL INFORMATION: 54

Portobello Mushrooms with Mediterranean Stuffing 56

INGREDIENTS: 56

DIRECTIONS: 57

Nutritional Information 58

Mediterranean Stuffed Tomatoes 60

INGREDIENTS: 60

DIRECTIONS: 61

Nutritional Information 61

reek Salmon Burgers 63

INGREDIENTS: 63

DIRECTIONS: 64

NutritionalInformation 64

Chicken-Garbanzo Salad 66

INGREDIENTS: 66

NutritionalInformation: 67

Two-Bean Greek Salad 69

INGREDIENTS 69

DIRECTIONS:.. 70

NutritionalInformation:.. 71

Stuffed Roasted Red Peppers 72

INGREDIENTS: 73

DIRECTIONS:.. 73

Nutritional Information:... 73

Mediterranean Basmati Salad 75

INGREDIENTS: 75

DIRECTIONS:.. 76

NutritionalInformation... 77

CHAPTER 4: DESSERTS **79**

RECIPES: 79

Almond Cake:... 79

INGREDIENTS: 80

DIRECTIONS:.. 80

Tiramisu 82

INGREDIENTS: 82

DIRECTIONS:.. 83

CRÈME CARAMEL 84

INGREDIENTS: 84

For the caramel:... 84

DIRECTIONS:.. 85

Orange and Hazelnut Cake with Orange Flower Syrup............ 86

INGREDIENTS- For the syrup 87

For the cake.. 87

To serve 87

DIRECTIONS:.. 87

Make the cake:.. 88

Toasted Bread with Chocolate: 89

INGREDIENTS: 90

DIRECTIONS:.. 90

CHAPTER 5: SNACKS **91**

RECIPES 91

Garlic Kale Hummus.. 91

INGREDIENTS: 91

DIRECTIONS:.. 92

Marinated Olives and Feta 93

INGREDIENTS: 93

DIRECTIONS: 94

NUTRITION 94

Lemon Basil Shrimp and Pasta 95

INGREDIENTS: 95

DIRECTIONS: 96

Artichoke and Arugula Pizza with Prosciutto 97

INGREDIENTS: 97

DIRECTIONS: 98

CONCLUSION **99**

The human brain is the single most magnificent miracle ever designed in the history of the universe. Weighing just 3 pounds, but demanding 25 percent of the blood from each heartbeat, your brain is the origin of every thought, emotion, movement, and dream.

Recently, neuroscience has taught us that our brains have "neural plasticity," which means they're dynamic and constantly reorganizing. We now know our brains can generate new brain cells (neurogenesis), and that environment and lifestyle can shape our brains. While we don't yet have a cure or even prevention for brain disease, we do have the ability to shape our brains for health—and it is never too early or late to get started.

I have studied the brain and behavior for more than 10 years, and my mission is to teach all humans, regardless of age or background, about this wonderful miracle that sits between our ears and how we all have the power to shape our brains for health throughout our lifespan. And with this easy- to-read and practical guide, you can get started.

The content of the book outlines this distinct pillar for brain health: *Smart Eating*

This is the area I've been emphasizing in my own work, too, because research has shown that it can make a difference. This book offers specific tips and Recipes that are easy and delicious too.

This book will add to the growing attention paid to brain health. Most important, by getting started today in one or more of these Delicious recipes, you are shaping your brain to be as healthy as it can be and maintaining access to your life story.

We Congratulate you for buying this book "Keep Sharp Recipes: Easy and Delicious Recipes to Help you Build a Better Brain at Any Age" Because you have made the best decision, knowing fully well that it is important to attend to your brain health at the earliest of ages.

Get started today on your journey to a Sharp & Healthy Brain.

Antioxidants! Omega-3s! Anti-inflammatory diets! Can something you eat really help you remember—again—where you put your cellphone or reading glasses? If you add blueberries to your morning oatmeal or sip a glass of red wine at dinner, will your brain cells stay healthier longer?

Much of what we hear about the interplay between diet and brain health is based on preliminary research and then flooded in hype. As headlines have linked one food or another to Alzheimer's disease and other illnesses, we have rushed to remove them from our diet. The problem is, as soon as one headline urges us to eat this, not that, it seems there's another saying just the opposite.

Why all the confusion? Proving conclusively which foods actually boost brain health is difficult and expensive, requiring large scale, long-term clinical trials. "When you're eating blueberries, you're not eating just one nutrient," explains Gene L.B, a brain nutrition researcher. "You're eating a complex mixture of hundreds of them. Is it the antioxidants that improved cognition or the vitamins? Most likely, it's the unique combination of all of them."

Still, it's become increasingly clear that how you eat may counteract the effects of an aging brain. "The best recipe is a diet that includes brain- building nutrients such as omega-3 fatty acids, antioxidants and certain vitamins, and steers clear of foods that promote high blood pressure, high cholesterol, obesity and diabetes," says Majid Fotuhi, M.D

It's never too late to start reaping the benefits of a brain-healthy diet. But don't try to detox all at once. Start slowly, and you'll soon realize that making more healthy choices isn't so hard after all.

Discover the 7 Secrets to a Healthy Brain and Keeping sharp. Here's what you need to know.

SECRET 1: GO MEDITERRANEAN.

A large body of very solid research shows that a classic "Mediterranean diet"—heavy in olive oil, legumes, fish, fruits and green leafy vegetables— protects against cardiovascular disease, diabetes and cancer. The link between the diet and brain health has been less conclusive—but that's changing. We have Prepared Great Recipes For you in This Book.

Some years ago, researchers at Columbia University in New York and the University of Miami Miller School of Medicine reported in *Archives of Neurology* that older adults who followed a Mediterranean diet had less of the kind of damage to the brain's small blood vessels that leads to a slowdown in mental quickness.

Previous studies by the same researchers found that the diet helped slow the onset of Alzheimer's disease, even in those who had only followed it occasionally.

In recent years, in reported the *New England Journal of Medicine*, Spanish scientists who had followed for five years more than 7,000 older adults at high risk for heart disease reported that those who ate a Mediterranean-style diet, including olive oil and a daily glass of red wine, showed about a 30 percent drop in heart attacks, strokes and deaths from heart disease, compared with a control group who ate more or less what they'd always eaten.

"As we age, the Mediterranean diet lowers the risk of

the strokes and ministrokes that lead to Alzheimer's pathology," says Rudolph E. T, M.D. "The rule of thumb," he says, is "what's good for your heart is good for your brain."

Tip

Go fish! Cold-water fatty fish are high in omega-3 fatty acids, a healthy fat linked to lower levels of beta-amyloid plaques (a sign of Alzheimer's). Omega-3s also boost the production of brain derived neurotrophic factor (BDNF), the protein that acts as fertilizer for the brain and is responsible for ramping up memory, mood and alertness.

Opt for a 4-ounce serving of salmon, Atlantic mackerel, sardines or herring, two or three times a week. But go light on fish that are high in mercury, such as king mackerel, bluefish and swordfish.

SECRET 2: RAMP UP FOODS RICH IN OMEGA-3S.

Your brain needs a certain amount of fat to function properly. Fats provide energy, help the body absorb essential vitamins and protect nerve cells and connections. But there are good and bad fats, and too much of the wrong kind throws a monkey wrench into the works, speeding the formation of beta-amyloid plaques.

Omega-3s are among the good fats. Research shows that they fight inflammation and support the structure of brain cells. A 2012 report in

Neurology by Gene Bowman's team at Oregon Health & Science University found that study participants (average age: 87) who had high blood levels of healthy fats, including omega-3s and a variety of vitamins (including B, C, D and E) and low levels of trans fats had less brain shrinkage and scored better on cognitive tests than those who ate less nutritious diets.

Tip

The body doesn't produce fatty acids naturally, so you must add them to your diet. If you're like most people, you are eating far too many inflammation-promoting omega-6 fatty acids and far too few omega-3s. What to do? In addition to eating more fish, add flaxseed to your cereal and smoothies and chia seeds to stir fries and salads. Both are stuffed with omega-3s (and have little taste). How much should you eat? According to the Cleveland Clinic, one to two tablespoons is a healthy daily dose.

SECRET 2: BINGE ON HEALTHY FRUITS

Binge on blueberries… as well as strawberries, spinach, kale and butternut squash.

Brightly colored fruits and dark green vegetables are rich in carotenoids and flavonoids—powerful antioxidants that boost BDNF, that brain derived neurotrophic factor mentioned earlier, and may slow the onset of dementia by repairing the damage from free radicals, unstable molecules that attack healthy cells.

Researchers at the Brigham and Women's Hospital in Boston found that older women who ate two or more servings of strawberries and blueberries a day were able to forestall memory decline by 2½ years. Green vegetables are also high in magnesium, a potent nutrient in the war against inflammation.

Tip

Aim for four to five servings a day of fruits and vegetables. Besides the ones mentioned above, try avocadoes, red grapes and raisins, raspberries, plums and prunes, spinach, beets, asparagus, sweet red peppers, sweet potatoes and citrus fruits.

If you take any medications, check with your doctor before adding to your diet grapefruit, which can cut the effectiveness of a host of drugs,

including many statins and antihistamines.

SECRET 4: CUT BACK ON RED MEAT AND DAIRY PRODUCTS.

Red meat is a good source of protein as well as essential vitamins and minerals, including B12, iron and zinc. But many cuts are high in unhealthy saturated fats, as are whole-milk dairy products. Saturated fats raise blood levels of the "bad" LDL cholesterol linked to heart disease and impaired memory. Harvard's Tanzi thinks the evidence to limit meat is strong: He's been a vegetarian for years.

Tip

If you can't live in a world without greasy cheeseburgers, indulge occasionally. Choose leaner cuts of beef, such as those with "loin" or "round" on the label, such as sirloin and round roast or steak. Avoid chuck. Other good sources of protein: beans and legumes, such as kidney beans, split peas and lentils. Nosh on an ounce a day of almonds, walnuts or cashews.

So many studies have shown a link between dementia and obesity and high blood sugar at midlife that Alzheimer's disease has been dubbed "diabetes Type 3." In 2012, Mayo Clinic scientists found that people age 70 and older who ate a lot of simple carbohydrates (found in refined flours and rice) and sugar were nearly four times more likely to develop mild cognitive impairment than those who ate a healthier diet.

Your body does need a certain amount of sugar (glucose) to function properly. But a diet packed with sugar and the simple carbs regularly sends blood glucose soaring. High glucose levels, in turn, block blood flow to the brain, depriving it of the energy it needs to generate new neurons. Too much glucose has also been implicated in the formation of the tangles of Alzheimer's disease.

Tip

You're already likely eating more sugar than you need,

since it's added to many beverages and foods during processing, so don't add it to your coffee or sprinkle it on already sweet fruits. Instead of sodas, sports drinks and sweetened coffee drinks, drink water. If you eat canned fruit, make sure the label says "in its own juice," not sugary syrup.

The easiest way to cut down on simple carbs is to opt for whole grain rice, breads and pastas. Whole grains are digested more slowly, so glucose also is released more slowly into the bloodstream, keeping you mentally alert longer. "Whole" or "whole grain" should appear on the label before the name of the grain.

Don't be fooled by phrases on labels that sound healthy but don't really mean much, such as "100 percent wheat," "cracked wheat," "multigrain" or "stone ground." Even better: Buy wheat berries, bulgur or faro—whole grains that haven't yet been ground into flour.

SECRET 6: TAKE THE SALTSHAKER OFF THE TABLE.

Doctors have warned for years that too much salt is bad for the heart. Now, a study by Canadian scientists has found that older people who eat too much salt and also fail to exercise are at increased risk for cognitive decline. According to the U.S. Department of Agriculture, if you are 50- plus, or suffer from high blood pressure, your salt intake should max out at no more than 1,500 milligrams a day.

Tip

Liven up your dishes with herbs and spices instead of processed gravies, condiments and sauces, which tend to be high in sodium. Many herbs and spices—including ginger, parsley, oregano, basil and black pepper—are not only flavorful but also high in antioxidants.

Curcumin, a key component of turmeric, found in curry powders, is believed to reduce amyloid plaque buildup. The brain benefits of these

SECRET 7: SLASH TRANS FATS.

Trans fats are processed fats added to foods to extend their shelf life. These fats are double trouble—they both raise blood levels of "bad" cholesterol and lower levels of "good" cholesterol.

Bowman's research suggests they are also bad for the brain. When his team members checked the blood levels of certain nutrients in 104 elderly participants, they found that those high in trans fats had significantly lower cognitive performance and less total brain volume than those who ate a healthier diet.

Tip

Buy and prepare fresh foods as often as possible. Packaged and processed foods are full of trans fats, so read labels and if you see "partially hydrogenated" anything, don't buy it. Common culprits: french fries, chips, packaged baked goods, crackers, icing, stick margarine (tub margarine has less trans fat) and microwave popcorn. If you can't or won't cut out foods with a lot of trans fat, eat less of them, and eat them less often.

CHAPTER 2: KEEP SHARP RECIPES

BREAKFAST

As with any other diet, breakfast is a very essential meal that can't be missed whatsoever. It does not always have to mean Greek yogurt parfaits. The basic principles of eating apply here also. This is where all the diets are similar because you need to have a proper filling meal that gives you the energy to keep going throughout the day. Below mentioned are a few recipes that you can add in order to make your breakfast very filling as well as full of variety, while being healthy also.

RECIPES

CHICK PEAS AND POTATO HASH

Eating Well's hash is a very good idea during any time of the idea but it has its specific benefits if you consider it for the breakfast. The best thing about it is that it will make you feel full and energetic enough to keep you going throughout the day. It contains 14 grams of protein, and 6 grams of fiber per serving. The quantity will be enough to serve 4 people at a time.

INGREDIENTS:

- 4 cups frozen shredded hash brown potatoes

- 2 cups finely chopped baby spinach

- ½ cup finely chopped onion

- 1 tablespoon minced fresh ginger

- 1 tablespoon curry powder

- ½ teaspoon salt

- ¼ cup extra-virgin olive oil

- 1 (15-ounce) can chickpeas, rinsed

- 1 cup chopped zucchini

- 4 large eggs

DIRECTIONS:

The directions for this recipe are very simple. All you have to do is: combine potatoes, spinach, onion, ginger, curry powder, and salt in a large bowl. Now take a large non-stick pan and heat some oil in it over a medium- high heat. Now add the potato mixture and press into a layer. Now make sure you cook without stirring for an approximate time of 3 to 5 minutes.

Keep on cooking until the potatoes become crispy and golden brown on the bottom. Now reduce the heat to a medium-low level. Fold in chickpeas and zucchini, and break the large chunks of potatoes until they are thoroughly combined. Now, press them back properly into another layer. Carve out 4 holes in the mixture.

Now break the eggs in such a way that one egg is broken at a time. Put them all in a cup and after mixing them, just pour them into each of the indentations. Now again cover the pan and keep on cooking until the eggs are set. In case you are interested in soft- set yolks, you should cook them for a maximum period of 4 to 5 minutes.

AVOCADO TOAST

Here we have another amazing recipe that will again lead you towards a very healthy life style. There is one thing that you need to take special care of. Make sure you pick a bread that is made up of whole grains for this breakfast. In Mediterranean diet, in order to make the food taste fresh, seasoning is done and large amounts of herbs are used which gives it a very refreshing taste and smell. In case you don't want to use bread then you can use rye as a substitute for the specific type of bread.   Below mentioned are the specific ingredients for the avocado toast.

INGREDIENTS:

- 2 small firm ripe avocados, that are peeled and seed is removed
- 80 grams soft feta which is crumbled
- 2 tablespoons chopped fresh mint, plus extra to garnish
- squeeze of fresh lemon juice, to taste
- 4 large slices rye bread

DIRECTIONS:

Place the avocado in a medium sized bowl and mash it roughly with a fork. Now add some mint to the mixture along with the squeeze of the lemon juice. Mix them properly until a homogeneous mixture is formed. Now that a thorough mixture has been prepared, season it with seas salt and freshly ground black pepper which is going to add to the taste and the flavor of the dish. Now coming towards the rye bread, toast it or grill it until it becomes golden in color. In order to serve, put 1/4th of the avocado mixture on each slice of the bread. In order to enhance the flavoring, top it with feta. If you want to give it a very fresh look then garnish it with extra mint. A very smart tip is to add some thinly shaved ham or you can even top it with a poached egg. Either way, your dish is going to both look as well as taste amazing.

MEDITERRANEAN FRITTATA

Eating vegetables for breakfast might not seem like a very appealing idea but if you add frittata to it then it will become good enough a recipe for breakfast. You can add a little bit of products to your beaked egg breakfast which is going to add to the flavor and the taste of the recipe. In this case you have an option of adding onions, red peppers and olives. Other than these, other varieties of peppers could also be added. It can serve 6 people at a time.

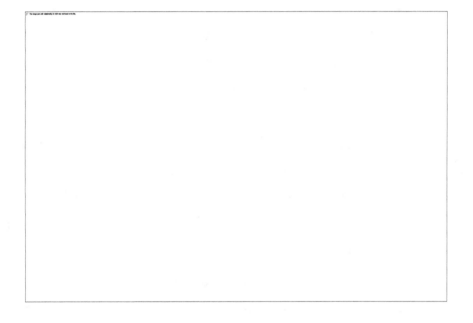

INGREDIENTS:

- 1 cup chopped onion
- 2 cloves minced garlic
- 3 tablespoons olive oil
- 8 eggs- beaten
- ¼ cup light cream or milk
- ½ cup crumbled feta cheese (2 ounces)
- ½ cup chopped bottled roasted red sweet peppers
- ½ cup sliced pitted ripe olives (optional)
- ¼ cup slivered fresh basil
- ⅛ teaspoon ground black pepper
- ½ cup onion and coarsely crushed garlic croutons
- 2 tablespoons finely shredded Parmesan cheese
- Fresh basil leaves (optional)0

DIRECTIONS:

The first step is to preheat the broiler. In a large skillet cook onion and garlic in approximately 2 table spoons of hot oil. Make sure you keep on heating it until onions become tender. While this part of cooking is in the process, you should simultaneously beat the eggs together in a bowl. Now that you have beaten the eggs properly, stir in some feta cheese and roasted sweet pepper.

You can add olives also but that is optional. You can add them if desired. After this, add some basil and black pepper. Now that a complete mixture is being prepared, pour it over the onion mixture that is being cooked in the skillet. After pouring it, cook it over a medium-heat flame. After heating for a little while the mixture will set. When this happens, run a spatula around the edge of the skillet so that the egg mixture is lifted and the uncooked portion flows underneath. Continue doing this until the egg mixture is completely set. You will realize that it is completely cooked when the surface gets little moist. Once this point is reached, just reduce the intensity of the flame in order to prevent over cooking. Now take another bowl and add crushed croutons, parmesan cheese and the remaining table spoons of oil. Sprinkle this mixture over the frittata. Make sure the top is set and the crumbs are golden. Cut this frittata in wedges and serve them right away. If you wish to garnish it then you can even do that with fresh basil leaves.

PANCAKES

Pancakes have always been one of the most delicious options for breakfast. You can alter their making a little and make them taste even better and healthier. What you have to do is; get some whole grains with your Greek yogurt and enjoy by making a stack of pancakes using the recipe.You can make a special topping with fresh fruits,toasted nuts, more Greek yogurt. You can even sweeten the stack with a dash of syrup. It makes about 6 servings.

INGREDIENTS:

- 1 cup old-fashioned oats
- ½ cup all-purpose flour
- 2 tablespoons flax seeds
- 1 teaspoon baking soda
- ¼ teaspoon salt
- 2 cups Greek yogurt (plain or vanilla)
- 2 large eggs
- 2 tablespoons agave or honey
- 2 tablespoons canola oil
- syrup, fresh fruit, or other toppings

DIRECTIONS:

Combine the first five ingredients in a blender and process them for 30 seconds. Add some yogurt, eggs, oil, and agave to it and again blend them until the mixture becomes really smooth. Let the batter stand for an approximate amount of 20 minutes so that it gets thickened. Batter can be prepared up to one day in advance. Just cover the batter and refrigerate. Heat the large non-stick skillet over medium heat. Brush the skillet with a small amount of oil. Ladle the batter in the skillet in such a way that ¼ of the cups are put in to it. The trick for cooking the pancakes is that keep on cooking them until bubbles are formed on the top and the bottom become golden brown. This is going to take 2 minutes at an average. Turn them over and again cook the other side also till it becomes golden brown. Transfer them to the baking sheet and keep them warm in the oven. Repeat the same process all over again with the remaining batter. While you are repeating the process, just make sure you brush the skillet with more butter, if necessary. You can serve it with whatever topping you desire. It can be fruits or syrup or anything that you desire.

MEDITERRANEAN BREAKFAST COUSCOUS

This recipe is generally not preferred for breakfast and is primarily considered for dinner but you can always change the classical recipes by making a few changes. By adding a little bit of brown sugar and dried fruit you can alter the classical dish and add whole grain to your Mediterranean diet. It is going to serve 4 people at a time.

INGREDIENTS:

- 3 cups of 1 percent low-fat milk
- 1 (2-inch) cinnamon stick
- 1 cup uncooked whole-wheat couscous
- ½ cup chopped dried apricots
- ¼ cup dried currants
- 6 teaspoons dark brown sugar
- ¼ teaspoon salt
- 4 teaspoons of melted and divided butter melted and divided

DIRECTIONS:

Combine milk and cinnamon stick in a large saucepan. Heat the mixture over a medium-high flame for approximately 3 minutes. Another indication for the cessation of heating is that when you start to see small bubbles from around inner edge of the pot then remove the source of heat. Make sure you do not boil it. Now that you have removed it from the stove, add couscous, apricots, currants and 4 tea spoons of brown sugar along with a small amount of salt. While adding these things, make sure you are constantly stirring.

Cover the mixture, and let it stand for 15 minutes. Remove and discard cinnamon stick. Divide the couscous in to four parts and put each one of them in one bowl so that you can top each one of them 1 tea spoon of melted butter and half a teas poon of brown sugar.

CHAPTER 3: LUNCH

Lunch is comparatively a lighter meal and should be regulated in such a way that there is a proper management of the calorie intake. You need to monitor your calorie intake more precisely for the lunch because that's the time when we eat a lot of other things like snacks etc also, other than the basic meal. Hence, below mentioned are a few recipes that will help you in deciding what you should have for lunch.

RECIPES:

MANGO AND BLACK BEAN SALAD:

Canned beans are a great item to add in the dishes if you want to have a certain cnetent if fiber and protein. This recipe is even more beneficial because it has mango and black beans in it without any salt in order to keep a check on the sodium levels. The good thing is that the sweet taste of mango neutralizes the earthiness of the beans and enhances their taste. You can even garnish it with fresh cilantro in order to make it look more appetizing. To give a more salivating effect, just serve it with spicy pork tender-loins.

INGREDIENTS:

- 1 and a 1/2 cups chopped peeled ripe mango
- 1 cup thinly sliced green onions
- 1/2 cup cooked wild or brown rice
- 3 tablespoons finely chopped fresh cilantro
- 2 tablespoons roasted tomatillo or fresh salsa
- 2 tablespoons fresh lime juice
- 2 tablespoons extravirgin olive oil
- 3/4 teaspoon salt
- 1/4 teaspoon freshly ground black pepper

- 1 (15-ounce) can organic no-salt-added black beans, rinsed and drained

All you have to do is- combine all ingredients in a large bowl. Toss gently to mix. This recipe contains a total of 334 calories.

CHICKEN, CARROT AND CUCUMBER SALAD:

The best way of serving this salad is by putting it in the plate with pita wedges or pita chips. You can either buy the pita chips or else

you can even make your own by spraying the pita wedges with cooking spray and sprinkle very small amounts of parmesan cheese that is shredded. Bake them for almost 10 minutes at a temperature of 400 degrees.

INGREDIENTS:

- 2 cups chopped cooked chicken breast
- 1 1/4 cups chopped seeded cucumber
- 1/2 cup matchstick-cut carrots
- 1/2 cup sliced radishes
- 1/3 cup chopped green onions
- 1/4 cup light mayonnaise
- 2 tablespoons chopped fresh cilantro
- 1 teaspoon bottled minced garlic
- 1/4 teaspoon salt
- 1/4 teaspoon ground cumin
- 1/8 teaspoon black pepper
- 4 green leaf lettuce leaves
- 4 (6-inch) whole wheat pitas, each cut into 8 wedges

DIRECTIONS:

Combine the chopped and cooked chicken breast along with chopped seeded cucumber, carrots, radishes, green onions in a large bowl.

Combine mayonnaise and fresh cilantro, minced garlic, salt, ground cumin and black pepper in another comparatively small bowl. Keep on stirring with a whisk.

Next step is to add the mayonnaise mixture to the chicken mixture and keep on stirring until they are properly mixed.Place 1 lettuce leaf on each of 4 plates; top each leaf with about 1 cup chicken mixture. Also, place 8 pita wedges with each serving plate. This recipe contains 382 calories.

MEDITERRANEAN PASTA SALAD

Mediterranean Pasta salad is an amazing choice as it contains only 420 calories per serving and has very negligible amounts of unsaturated fats.

INGREDIENTS:

- 8 ounces multigrain farfalle
- Zest and juice of 1 lemon
- 2 teaspoons olive oil
- 1 13.5- ounce can artichoke hearts packed in water, drained and chopped
- 8 ounces fresh part- chopped skim mozzarella cheese
- 1/4 cup chopped bottled roasted red bell pepper
- 1/4 cup chopped fresh parsley
- 1/2 cup frozen peas

DIRECTIONS:

While cooking pasta, make sure you follow the instructions that are being provided on the package. Don't forget to get rid of the salt and fat. While your pasta is on the stove, combine the juice of 1 lemon and two teaspoons of olive oil in a large bowl. Make sure you stir it well with a whisk. Now add bell pepper, cheese, artichoke hearts and parsley and toss it to mix well.

Next step is to place peas in a colander and right after the pasta is cooked drain pasta over peas. Shake them wellto drain properly but do not run under cold water at al. now the job is almost done and all you have to do is; add pasta and peas to artichoke mixture and toss well until the mixture is thoroughly combined. Serve warm or at room temperature depending upon your liking.

MEDITERRANEAN CHICKPEA PATTIES

The good thing about chick pea patties is that they are very easy to make because the total time period of preparing as well as cooking it is 20 minutes in total. They have very less number of calories in them; only 225 calories per serving.

INGREDIENTS:

- 1 (15.5-ounce) can chickpeas, rinsed and drained
- 1/2 cup fresh flat-leaf parsley
- 1 chopped garlic clove
- 1/4 teaspoon ground cumin
- 1/2 teaspoon divided kosher salt
- 1/2 teaspoon divided black pepper
- 1 whisked egg
- 4 tablespoons all-purpose flour
- 2 tablespoons olive oil
- 1/2 cup low-fat Greek-style yogurt
- 3 tablespoons fresh lemon juice
- 8 cups mixed salad greens
- 1 cup grape tomatoes, halved
- 1/2 small thinly sliced red onion
- Pita chips (optional)

DIRECTIONS:

Pulse chick peas, flat-leaf parsley, garlic clove and cumin along with ¼ tea spoon of salt and pepper both, in a food processor until a viscous chopped mixture comes out now transfer this mixture to a bowl. Now add an egg and two table spoons of flour to the already prepared mixture. Make around 8 roll patties out of this mixture. Each patty should be approximately ½ inch thick. Do not waste the remaining flour. Put it in a small dish and roll the patties in it with the floured hands. To give it a neat look, tap off the excess flour. Now that you are done with the preparatory phase of the recipe, next up is the cooking phase.

First of all heat the oil in a non-stick skillet over a medium-high flame. Cook the patties from each side for an approximate amount of 2-3 minutes, until they turn a little golden in color. Now whisk some lemon juice and yogurt together and add the remaining salt and pepper to it.

Put the garnishing stuff beautifully on the plate which should include green lettuce and tomatoes and onions. You can add other things also, depending upon your own choice. Sprinkle the salad with 2 table spoons of the dressing. Serve with pita chips if you feel like it.

MEDITERRANEAN SHRIMP AND PASTA

Shrimps are an all-time favorite of all the food lovers and a combination of both pasta and shrimps is very salivating when you even think about it. For calorie conscious people it is a very good idea because it only contains 424 calories per serving.

INGREDIENTS:

- 2 teaspoons olive oil
- Cooking spray
- 2 minced garlic cloves
- 1 pound peeled and deveined medium shrimp
- 2 cups chopped plum tomato
- 1/4 cup thinly sliced fresh basil
- 1/3 cup chopped pitted kalamata olives
- 2 tablespoons drained capers
- 1/4 teaspoon freshly ground black pepper
- 4 cups hot cooked angel hair pasta (about 8 ounces uncooked pasta)
- 1/4 cup (2 ounces) crumbled feta cheese

DIRECTIONS:

First of all take small quantity of olive oil and heat olive oil in a large nonstick skillet which is coated with the cooking spray. Heat it over a medium-high flame. Now the next step is to add garlic and sauté it for 30 seconds. Secondly add shrimp and again sauté for one minute. Third step is to add tomato and basil. After you have done that, reduce the heat of the flame and simmer 3 minutes or at least until the tomato is tender. When the tomato is tender enough- stir in some kalamata olives and capers along with black pepper. The last and the most important step would be the combination of the shrimp mixture and pasta. Combine these two in a large bowl and toss the mixture well. Top it with cheese in order to give a delicious taste and texture to the recipe.

MEDITERRANEAN PIZZA

In case you are a pizza fan, this recipe is the best recipe for you because it contains as less as 291 calories and is extremely easy to make because it takes only 17 minutes to get ready, including the preparatory time.

INGREDIENTS:

- 1 (12-inch) prepared pizza crust
- 1/4 teaspoon crushed red pepper
- 1/4 teaspoon dried Italian seasoning
- 1 cup (4 ounces) crumbled goat cheese
- 3 sliced plum tomatoes (1/4-inch-thick slices)
- 6 chopped pitted kalamata olives
- 1 (14-ounce) can of drained quartered artichoke hearts
- Cooking spray
- 1/4 cup chopped fresh basil or 4 teaspoons dried basil

DIRECTIONS:

First of all preheat the oven to 450° temperature before you start doing any other thing. Now sprinkle the pizza crust with crushed red pepper and dried Italian seasoning. Spread the crumbled goat cheese evenly on the crust, leaving approximately a 1/2-inch border. Now in order to get a smooth surface just press the cheese down on the pizza crust gently with the back of the spoon.

Now that is up to you that what kind of arrangement you want for the top of the pizza. You can arrange the plum tomato slices, chopped olives, and quartered artichoke hearts on the pizza in whatever pattern you desire. Now place this pizza on a baking sheet which is properly coated with the cooking spray.

Bake the pizza for approximately 10-12 minutes. Make sure you bake it till the crust is crisp and the cheese is soft and bubbly. Now lastly, sprinkle the chopped basil over the top and serve the delicious and hot pizza. Enjoy the best flavors with the right kind of calorie-intake.

Dinner is an equally important meal of the day. Most of us tend to be very careless about the dinner and think that this meal can be skipped. This is a very mal practice and should be discontinued altogether. It is very important to have at least something for the dinner. In case you are worried about what you should have for the dinner because you don't want to gain any extra fat then don't worry about it at all because we have it all sorted out here. the recipes mentioned below will provide you with the most amazing low calorie based foods that are going to taste amazing as well.

RECIPES:

MEDITERRANEAN SEA- FOOD GRILL WITH SKORDALIA

This is an amazing recipe for all the sea-food lovers and we have also mentioned the whole nutrition chart for you so that you get to know the nutritional value of all these recipes as well.

INGREDIENTS:

- 1 pound russet or Yukon gold potatoes
- 8 peeled garlic cloves
- 1 slice sourdough bread with the crust removed
- 1/4 cup plain Greek low-fat yogurt
- 3 tablespoons olive oil
- Zest and juice of 1 lemon
- 1/2 teaspoon salt

- 1/4 teaspoon dried thyme
- 1 pound halibut fillets cut into 4 pieces
- 2 quartered red bell peppers
- 1 pound small zucchini diagonally cut into 1-inch pieces
- 1/2 sliced red onions

DIRECTIONS:

Firstly, peel the potatoes and chop them in such a way that the pieces are approximately one inch each. Place the potatoes in a large saucepan and cover them with cold water. Now in order to add flavor, add garlic and cook over high heat flame for an approximate time of 15 minutes or to get an easier idea cook them until the potatoes are easily pierced with a fork. While the potatoes cook, tear the bread into 3 or 4 pieces and place it in a large bowl.

Take almost 3 to 4 table spoons of the cooking liquid from the potatoes and pour it over the bread. Stir it with a fork until it becomes really smooth. Now add 2 tablespoons of yogurt and olive oil. Also, add some zest and squeeze the juice of 1 lemon. Again stir it until a smooth paste is formed.

When potatoes are done you need to place a large bowl in the sink and set a colander on top. Drain the mixture of the potatoes and garlic while reserving the cooking liquid. Transfer the drained potatoes to bread mixture and mash until it become really smooth (a potato ricer works well for this task). Add the remaining cooking liquid in such a way that you must not add more than 2 tablespoons at a time. Keep adding until the mixture takes on the consistency of loose mashed potatoes. Add ½ teaspoon of salt and 2 teaspoons of olive oil. Cover and keep it warm until it is ready to serve. Preheat the grill pan over medium-high heat flame.

Drizzle fish with 1½ teaspoon of olive oil and season with remaining 1½ teaspoon of salt and thyme. Cook the fish for 2 to 3 minutes on each side until fish flakes are seen when it is tested with a fork or until desired degree of cooking is being done. Transfer it to a plate and then cover and keep warm until it is ready to serve. Place bell pepper, zucchini, and red onion in a large bowl. Sprinkle the remaining 1½ teaspoon olive oil and toss it to coat properly.

Arrange bell pepper in grill pan and cook for 5 minutes over medium-heat flame. Add zucchini and onion and cook for 10 minutes or until vegetables are tender. Keep on turning as necessary in order to make sure that the vegetables are evenly cooked.

NUTRITIONAL INFORMATION:

Calories per serving:	390
Fat per serving:	14g
Saturated fat per serving:	2g

Monounsaturated fat per serving: 8g

Polyunsaturated fat per serving: 2g

Protein per serving: 31g

Carbohydrates per serving: 37g

Fiber per serving: 5g

Cholesterol per serving: 35mg

Sodium per serving: 280mg

Resistant starch per serving: 1.7g

PORTOBELLO MUSHROOMS WITH MEDITERRANEAN STUFFING

Mushrooms are again a very good choice for the dinner and the reason why they are added here in this list is because we want you to have a variety of options that you can consider for dinner.

INGREDIENTS:

- 4 (4-inch) portobello caps (about 3/4 pound)
- 1/4 cup finely chopped onion
- 1/4 cup finely chopped celery
- 1/4 cup finely chopped carrot
- 1/4 cup finely chopped red bell pepper

- 1/4 cup finely chopped green bell pepper
- 1/4 teaspoon dried Italian seasoning
- 2 minced garlic cloves
- cooking spray
- 3 cups (1/4-inch) cubed toasted French bread, toasted
- 1/2 cup vegetable broth
- 1/2 cup (2 ounces) crumbled feta cheese
- 3 tablespoons low-fat balsamic vinaigrette
- 4 teaspoons grated fresh Parmesan cheese
- 1/4 teaspoon black pepper
- 4 cups mixed salad greens

DIRECTIONS:

Firstly, before starting anything else you must preheat the oven to 350°. Eradicate the stems from the mushrooms and finely chop stems to measure 1/4 cup. You can discard or keep the remaining stems and use them for some other purpose, depends on you. Combine 1/4 cup chopped stems, onion, celery, carrot, red bell pepper, green bell pepper and Italian seasoning.

Heat a large nonstick skillet over medium heat and before eating; coat the pan with cooking spray. Add the onion mixture to the pan and cook for 10 minutes or at leastthe until vegetables are tender enough. Combine the onion mixture and bread in a large bowl and toss it to combine. Slowly add the broth to the bread mixture and toss it to coat properly. Add feta and toss gently.Remove brown gills from the undersides of mushroom caps using a spoon and then discard the gills later on. Place mushrooms in such a way that the stem side should be up. Place them on a baking sheet which is coated with the cooking spray.

Brush the mushrooms evenly with 1 tablespoon of vinaigrette. Sprinkle Parmesan and black pepper evenly over the mushrooms and then top each with 1/2 cup bread mixture. Bake the mushrooms for 25 minutes at 350 degrees or at least until the mushrooms are tender.

Combine the remaining 2 tablespoons of vinaigrette and greens while tossing them gently. Place 1 cup of greens that you have kept for garnishing, on the plate and top the serving with 1 mushroom.

NUTRITIONAL INFORMATION

Calories per serving: 182

Calories from fat: 32%

Fat per serving: 6.4g

Saturated fat per serving: 3.5g

Monounsaturated fat per serving: 1.3g

Polyunsaturated fat per serving: 0.5g

Protein per serving: 9.3g

Carbohydrates per serving: 22.7g

Fiber per serving: 4.1g

Cholesterol per serving: 20mg

Iron per serving: 2.2mg

Sodium per serving: 691mg

Calcium per serving: 189mg

MEDITERRANEAN STUFFED TOMATOES

INGREDIENTS:

- 2 large tomatoes
- 1/2 cup packaged garlic croutons
- 1/4 cup (1 ounce) crumbled goat cheese
- 1/4 cup sliced pitted kalamata olives
- 2 tablespoons reduced-fat vinaigrette or Italian salad dressing
- 2 tablespoons chopped fresh thyme or basil

DIRECTIONS:

Firstly preheat the broiler and then cut the tomatoes in half crosswise. Use your finger to push out and discard the seeds. Make sure you use a paring knife to cut out the pulp. You should leave two shells. Then chop the pulp and transfer to a medium bowl. Place the hollowed tomatoes and cut the sides down on a paper towel. Drain for 5 minutes.

Add croutons, goat cheese, olives, dressing, and thyme or basil to pulp and mix them well. Put the mixture into the hollowed tomatoes. Place those tomatoes on a baking sheet or a broiler pan. Broil 4-5 inches from heat until hot and cheese melts for approximately 5 minutes and then in order to get the best taste just serve immediately.

NUTRITIONAL INFORMATION

Calories per serving: 103

Fat per serving: 7g

Saturated fat per serving: 2g

Monounsaturated fat per serving: 3g

Polyunsaturated fat per serving: 0.5g

Protein per serving: 3g

Carbohydrates per serving: 8g

Fiber per serving: 1g

Cholesterol per serving: 6mg

Iron per serving: 1mg

Sodium per serving: 303mg

Calcium per serving: 39mg

REEK SALMON BURGERS

INGREDIENTS:

- 1 pound skinless salmon fillets, cut into 2-inch pieces
- 1/2 cup panko
- 1 large egg white
- 1 pinch kosher salt
- 1/4 teaspoon freshly ground black pepper

- 1/2 cup cucumber slices
- 1/4 cup crumbled feta cheese
- 4 (2.5-oz) ciabatta rolls, toasted

DIRECTIONS:

Take a food processor and in its bowl, pulse salmon, panko, and egg white until salmon is finely chopped. Form salmon into 4 (4-inch) patties and season it with salt and pepper. Heat the grill to medium-high flame and cook while turning once until burgers are just cooked thoroughly. This will take 5-7 minutes per side. Serve it with desired toppings and buns.

NUTRITIONAL INFORMATION

Calories per serving: 443

Fat per serving: 12.8g

Saturated fat per serving: 3.4g

Monounsaturated fat per serving: 3.4g

Polyunsaturated fat per serving: 3.4g

Protein per serving: 36g

Carbohydrates per serving: 42g

Fiber per serving: 1g

Cholesterol per serving: 84mg

Iron per serving: 3mg

Sodium per serving: 655mg

Calcium per serving: 88mg

CHICKEN-GARBANZO SALAD

INGREDIENTS:

- 1 (9-ounce) package frozen cooked chopped chicken breast
- 1 (15-ounce) rinsed and drained can chickpeas (garbanzo beans)
- 1 cup chopped seeded cucumber (about 1 small)
- 1/2 cup chopped green onions (about 4 small)

- 1/4 cup chopped fresh mint or basil
- 1/2 cup plain fat-free yogurt
- 2 minced garlic cloves
- 1/4 teaspoon salt
- 2 cups prepackaged baby spinach leaves
- 1/3 cup (1.3 ounces) feta cheese with cracked pepper
- 4 lemon wedges

All you have to do is- combine the first 8 ingredients and toss them gently. Gently fold in spinach leaves and feta cheese. Serve the salad with lemon wedges. So easy to make and even easier to serve!

NUTRITIONALINFORMATION:

Calories per serving:	258g
Calories from fat:	21%
Fat per serving:	6g
Saturated fat per serving:	2.7g
Monounsaturated fat per serving:	1.6g
Polyunsaturated fat per serving:	1g

Protein per serving: 27.8g

Carbohydrates per serving: 22.9g

Fiber per serving: 4.9g

Cholesterol per serving: 66mg

Iron per serving: 2.9mg

Sodium per serving: 675mg

Calcium per serving: 190mg

TWO-BEAN GREEK SALAD

INGREDIENTS

- 2 tablespoons red wine vinegar
- 2 teaspoons Dijon mustard
- 3 teaspoons chopped fresh oregano
- 4 1/2 teaspoons olive oil

- 1/2 teaspoon freshly ground black pepper
- 1 (10-ounce) bag shelled frozen edamame or lima beans
- 3/4 pound string beans
- 1 cup halved grape tomatoes
- 1/4 cup pitted kalamata olives, halved
- 2 multigrain pitas, halved horizontally
- 3 ounces haloumi cheese (or ricotta salata), sliced into 4 pieces

DIRECTIONS:

In a serving bowl, whisk together red wine vinegar, Dijon mustard, 2 1/2 teaspoons oregano, 2 teaspoons olive oil, and 1/4 teaspoon pepper and set them aside. Place the steamer basket in saucepan filled with a few inches of water and cook edamame which needs to stay covereduntil it gets tender which is going to be approximately 3 minutes. Transfer this edamame to a bowl and add string beans to steamer.

Cook them properly and again keep them covered until they become tender which means approximately 2 minutes. Now is the time to add beans to edamame. Add tomatoes and olives also and again toss to mix them. Now that you are done with the initial steps, heat a lightly oiled grill pan over medium-high flame and brush 1 teaspoon oil on one side of pitas; grill it and keep turning until it turns golden. This is going to take approximately 2 minutes.

Transfer pitas to a plate. Again brush 1/2 teaspoon oil evenly on one side of cheese slices and sprinkle it with the remaining oregano and pepper. Grill cheese in such a way that the seasoned side is facing down. Keep on doing that until marks form which means almost a minute and transfer it to a plate. Place 1 pita and top it with bean salad and cheese. Drizzle with remaining olive oil.

NUTRITIONALINFORMATION:

Calories per serving: 301

Fat per serving: 17g

Saturated fat per serving: 5g

Monounsaturated fat per serving: 7g

Polyunsaturated fat per serving: 2g

Protein per serving: 16g

Carbohydrates per serving: 23g

Fiber per serving: 8g

Cholesterol per serving: 14mg

Iron per serving: 3mg

Sodium per serving: 519mg

Calcium per serving: 139mg

STUFFED ROASTED RED PEPPERS

INGREDIENTS:

- 6 large red bell peppers
- 1 tablespoon olive oil
- 4 minced garlic cloves
- 6 ounces fresh spinach
- 1 tablespoon fresh lemon juice
- 1 teaspoon salt
- 3/4 cup uncooked couscous (about 2 cups cooked)
- 1/2 cup crumbled feta cheese

DIRECTIONS:

The directions are really simple. All you have to do is just take the seeds out of the peppers and stuff them with the mixture formed by the combination of the above mentioned ingredients and then roast them.

NUTRITIONAL INFORMATION:

Calories per serving:216

Fat per serving: 8g

Saturated fat per serving: 4g

Monounsaturated fat per serving: 3g

Polyunsaturated fat per serving: 1g

Protein per serving: 9g

Carbohydrates per serving: 30g

Fiber per serving: 5g

Cholesterol per serving: 21mg

Iron per serving: 2mg

Sodium per serving: 479mg

Calcium per serving: 165mg

MEDITERRANEAN BASMATI SALAD

The image and/with relationship ID 1688 was not found in the file.

INGREDIENTS:

- 2 sun-dried tomatoes, packed without oil
- 1/4 cup hot water
- 1 1/4 cups uncooked basmati rice
- 2 cups water
- 1/2 teaspoon salt

- 2/3 cup (2.5 ounces) feta cheese, crumbled
- 2 tablespoons dried currants
- 2 tablespoons chopped fresh mint
- 1 tablespoon olive oil
- 1/4 teaspoon black pepper
- 2 tablespoons toasted pine nuts

DIRECTIONS:

Combine tomatoes and water in a small bowl and let it stand for 10 minutes. Drain and chop and then set aside.Place the rice in a large bowl and cover with water to 2 inches above rice. Soak for 30 minutes while stirring occasionally. Now again drain and rinse.Combine the rice and 2 cups of water in a small saucepan and then slowly stir in some salt.

Bring to a boil over medium-high flame while stirring frequently. Boil for 5 minutes or until water level falls just below the level of the rice. Cover it and then reduce the heat to low and cook for 10 minutes. Remove from heat and let it stand, again covered for 10 minutes. Spoon the rice into a bowland let them cool completely and then fluff them with a fork.

After you are done doing this, stir in some tomatoes, feta, and the next 4 ingredients and toss them well to combine. Sprinkle with pine nuts.

NUTRITIONALINFORMATION

Calories per serving: 358

Calories from fat: 29%

Fat per serving: 11.7g

Saturated fat per serving: 4.8g

Monounsaturated fat per serving: 4.7g

Polyunsaturated fat per serving: 1.7g

Protein per serving: 10g

Carbohydrates per serving: 57g

Fiber per serving: 1g

Cholesterol per serving: 22mg

Iron per serving: 1mg

Sodium per serving: 609mg

Calcium per serving: 142m

CHAPTER 4: DESSERTS

The desserts are the most important part of any meal and as they are taken at the end, they must be really delicious so that you can enjoy the after-taste of your meal. The more important fact is that the maximum numbers of calories are usually always present in the desserts due to the kind of ingredients that we use in them. Hence here is the list of the Mediterranean desserts that you can consume and not gain a lot of weight.

RECIPES:

ALMOND CAKE:

This is a delicious cake. Pilgrims and tourists see the cake in the windows of every pastry shop and restaurant. You must try it and see how amazing it tastes.

INGREDIENTS:

- 1/2 lb. (1-3/4 cups) blanched whole almonds
- 6 separated large eggs
- 1-1/4 cups superfine sugar
- Grated zest of 1 orange
- Grated zest of 1 lemon
- 4 drops almond extract
- Confectioners' sugar for dusting

DIRECTIONS:

Finely grind the almonds in a food processor. Then take an electric mixer and beat the egg yolks with the sugar to a smooth pale cream. Beat in the zests and almond extract also. Add the ground almonds and mix them very thoroughly. Take a clean beater and with that, beat the egg whites in a large bowl until stiff and hard peaks are formed. Fold them into the egg and almond mixture.

Bear this in mind that the mixture is very thick, so you will need to turn it over quite a bit into the egg whites. Take a non-stick pan and make sure it is at least 11inch in size and grease it with butter first and then dust it with flour. Pour in the cake batter, and bake in a preheated 350°F oven for 40 minutes. Bake it until it feels firm to the touch. Let it cool before turning out.Just to add to the flavor, right before serving, dust the top of the cake with confectioners' sugar.

TIRAMISU

This simple tiramisu recipe with rum is coffee-rich but still light and airy. It makes as a very impressive dessert that is also very incredibly amazing in taste.

INGREDIENTS:

- 360 ml very strong coffee, warm, or 6 double espressos
- 4 table spoon dark rum
- 250 g caster sugar
- 6 free-range medium eggs

- 120 ml marsala
- 500 g mascarpone
- 4 sponge fingers
- Cocoa powder for dusting

DIRECTIONS:

First of all, combine the coffee with the rum and 50g of the sugar. Stir the mixture until the sugar has dissolved and set aside. Separate the eggs and reserve the yolks in a large bowl. Take another clean bowl and whisk the whites until they are stiff. Add the remaining amount of the sugar and marsala to the yolks. Whisk until they are pale and fluffy and then add the mascarpone and gently stir it in.

Fold the whisked whites into the yolk mixture. Use 2 sponge fingers per glass. Dip each one in the coffee mixture in such a way that let it absorb enough of liquid to wet the whole finger without it breaking. Place half a finger at the bottom of a small glass tumbler (150ml). Spoon over a tablespoon of the mascarpone cream and then add the other half sponge finger and add another tablespoon of mascarpone cream. Sprinkle over a little cocoa powder and take another soaked sponge finger, break it in two and lay both halves on top, covering them with a little more of the cream.

Cover and place in the fridge for no fewer than 8 hours, or at least until properly set. At the end, dust the top of the pots with cocoa powder to serve.

CRÈME CARAMEL

INGREDIENTS:

- 4 eggs
- 1 egg yolk
- 120 g caster sugar
- 500 ml milk
- 1 drop vanilla essence

FOR THE CARAMEL:

- 150 g caster sugar

- 50 ml water

DIRECTIONS:

Preheat the oven to 140°C/gas 1. Whisk the whole eggs, egg yolk and sugar together in a bowl and then mix in the milk and vanilla essence. Pass the mixture through a fine sieve into a clean bowl. In order to make the caramel, boil the sugar and water together in a small pan without stirring until the syrup thickens and caramelizes. It needs to turn golden brown. Now pour the hot caramel into 4 moulds and then you should pour the egg mixture into each caramel-filled mould.

Place the carioles in a roasting tray and pour hot water in around the moulds until it reaches half-way up the side of the moulds. Next step is this that you should bake the crème caramels in the preheated oven for 40 minutes and after baking it for 40 minutes, remove it and set aside to cool. In order to serve, turn out of the moulds on to the serving plates.

ORANGE AND HAZELNUT CAKE WITH ORANGE FLOWER SYRUP

This is a wheat-free cake which is very light and fluffy and is soaked in a zesty syrup. Cakes are not as popular as filo pastries in the Eastern Mediterranean, but this is a specialty of the Jewish quarter on the Asian side of Istanbul.

INGREDIENTS- FOR THE SYRUP

- 1-1/4 cups superfine sugar
- 2-1/2 Tbs. orange juice
- 2-1/2 Tbs. orange flower water
- Grated zest of 1 orange

FOR THE CAKE

- 5 large eggs
- 1 cup superfine sugar
- 2-1/4 cups hazelnut flour or meal

TO SERVE

- 1-1/3 cups Greek-style yogurt
- 2 Tbs. confectioners' sugar
- Pulp of 4 passion fruits

DIRECTIONS:

Just like any other cake baking, preheat the oven to 350°F. Make the syrup in a saucepan.First of all bring 2/3 cup water to a boil. Then add the sugar and orange juice and simmer for 10 to 12 minutes until the sugar has dissolved and the mixture is thick and syrupy. Once it has reached this stage, remove from the heat and let it cool. Stir in the orange flower water and orange zest.

MAKE THE CAKE:

Beat the egg yolks in a bowl with the help of an electric mixer on a very high speed with the sugar until the mixture becomes thick and pale. Fold the hazelnut flour into the yolk mixture. In a separate bowl, whisk the egg whites until they become stiff and their appearance becomes a little glossy. Then gently fold them into the hazelnut mixture.Grease the loaf pan and line with parchment paper. Pour in the batter. Bake for about 30 minutes until they become lightly golden. Remove the cake from the oven and evenly pour the cooled orange syrup over the top. Before serving, combine the yogurt, confectioners' sugar and passion fruit pulp in a bowl and serve with the warm cake.

TOASTED BREAD WITH CHOCOLATE:

INGREDIENTS:

- 8 1/2-inch-thick slices good bread
- Best-quality extra-virgin olive oil for drizzling
- 4 oz. best-quality bittersweet chocolate, very coarsely chopped (scant 1 cup)
- Sea salt
- kosher salt or any specialty salt

DIRECTIONS:

Position a rack 4 inches from the broiler element and heat it to a high temperature. Put the bread on a baking sheet and toast until it becomes light golden on both sides. This will take 1 to 2 minutes per side. Drizzle the bread with olive oil. Distribute the chocolate evenly on top of the bread.

Turn off the broiler and return the bread to the oven until the residual heat melts the chocolate. This should not take more than 1 minute. Smooth the chocolate with a table knife, if you want. Sprinkle a pinch of salt on each slice and serve.

Snacks are amazing option for your mid-night cravings as well as for the daily routine munching. Below mentioned are some of the best Mediterranean snacks that you can make and enjoy them at any time of the day.

RECIPES

GARLIC KALE HUMMUS

INGREDIENTS:

- 2 Cup Cooked Chickpeas
- 1 Cup Torn and Washed Kale
- 1/2 Teaspoon Fresh Chopped Garlic
- 1/2 Teaspoon Onion Powder
- 1/4 Teaspoon Black Pepper
- 1/4Cup Water

DIRECTIONS:

Combine chickpeas, Kale, Spices, and Water into a blender or food processor and then blend it until it becomes a smooth mixture. Let it chill in the fridge and store in an airtight container for about 1 week.

MARINATED OLIVES AND FETA

INGREDIENTS:

- 1 cup sliced pitted olives, such as Kalamata or mixed Greek
- 1/2 cup diced feta cheese, preferably reduced-fat
- 2 tablespoons extra-virgin olive oil
- Zest and juice of 1 lemon
- 2 cloves sliced garlic
- 1 teaspoon chopped fresh rosemary
- Pinch of crushed red pepper
- Freshly ground pepper

DIRECTIONS:

Combine olives, feta, oil, lemon zest and juice, garlic, rosemary, crushed red pepper and black pepper in a medium bowl and then cover and refrigerate for up to 1 day.Olives and feta marinated with rosemary, lemon and garlic are great served on crisp flatbread-style crackers or warm slices of crusty baguette

NUTRITION

Per 2-tablespoonserving:

73 calories
7 g fat

6 mg cholesterol

2 g carbohydrate

0 g added sugars

1 g protein

0 g fiber

263 mg sodium

14 mg potassium.

LEMON BASIL SHRIMP AND PASTA

INGREDIENTS:

- 3 quarts water
- 8 ounces uncooked spaghetti
- 1 pound peeled and deveined large shrimp

- 1/4 cup chopped fresh basil
- 3 tablespoons drained capers
- 2 tablespoons olive oil
- 2 tablespoons fresh lemon juice
- 1/2 teaspoon salt
- 2 cups baby spinach

DIRECTIONS:

What you have to do is: bring 3 quarts of water to a boil in an oven. Add pasta and cook it for approximately 8 minutes. Now add shrimp to the pan and cook it for 3 minutes or until shrimp are done and pasta looks cooked enough. Drain it and place the pasta mixture in a large bowl. Stir in some basil and 3 table spoons of the drained capers and 2 table spoons of the olive oil. Add two table spoons of the fresh lemon juice also, along with the half tea spoon of salt. Place 1/2 cup spinach on the plate and top each serving with 1 1/2 cups pasta mixture.

ARTICHOKE AND ARUGULA PIZZA WITH PROSCIUTTO

A balance of flavors is the key to this recipe. The bitter arugula, sweet artichoke, salty prosciutto, and creamy mozzarella are in perfect equilibrium atop a crisp-and-chewy crust and pesto sauce. Not only is the combination of tastes more satisfying than pepperoni and red sauce but also this pizza takes just 11 minutes to bake—no longer than a frozen one. So isn't this an amazing option that you are getting here.

INGREDIENTS:

- Cooking spray
- 1 tablespoon cornmeal
- 1 (13.8-ounce) can refrigerated pizza crust dough
- 2 tablespoons commercial pesto
- 1/2 cup (2 ounces) shredded part-skim mozzarella cheese

- 1 (9-ounce) package frozen artichoke hearts, thawed and drained
- 1 ounce thinly sliced prosciutto
- 2 tablespoons shredded Parmesan cheese
- 1 1/2 cups arugula leaves
- 1 1/2 tablespoons fresh lemon juice

DIRECTIONS:

First and the foremost thing that you need to do is to position the oven rack to lowest setting. And then like any other baking recipe, you have to preheat the oven to a temperature of 500°. Now, coat a baking sheet with cooking spray and sprinkle it with cornmeal. Unroll the dough onto the prepared baking sheet, and pat into a 14 x 10-inch rectangle. Now make sure you spread the pesto evenly over the dough, leaving a 1/2-inch border. Next step is to sprinkle mozzarella cheese over pesto. Place the baking sheet on the bottom oven rack and bake at 500° for minimum 5 minutes. After that, remove the pizza from oven. Coarsely chop the artichokes. Arrange artichokes on pizza and top with sliced prosciutto. Sprinkle with Parmesan.

Return pizza to the bottom oven rack and now bake an additional 6 minutes or until the crust is browned. Now place arugula in a bowl and drizzle juice over arugula and toss gently. Top the pizza with arugula mixture. Cut the pizza into 4 (7 x 5-inch) rectangles and cut each rectangle diagonally into 2 wedges.

CONCLUSION

You pop a chicken in the oven to roast, call your sister about a graduation gift for your niece and—yikes!—you did it again. That unmistakable burnt- to-a-crisp smell is yet another sign that you can't remember anything anymore. To say you're worried is a serious understatement. Spacey moments happen to all of us, no matter how old we are. But when they happen at midlife, we panic.

Memory loss is a frightening thing. If you're worried about brain health, you're not alone. Research shows that Americans 50 and older are concerned about losing mental capacity. Infact, Staying mentally sharp is a top concern For most Americans.

Relax. "The truth is, 80 percent of people over 70 do not have significant memory loss," says Rudolph T, Ph.D.

And now many experts believe you can prevent or at least delay that decline—even if you have a genetic predisposition to dementia. Reducing Alzheimer's risk factors like obesity, diabetes, smoking and low physical activity by just 25 percent could prevent up to half a million cases of the disease in the United States, according to a recent analysis from the University of California in San Francisco. There's hope even for those senior moments.

We Believe this Vital Information we have provided for you and these delicious recipes will help to improve your Brain Health. Live Smart and Keep Sharp.

We Recommend you to Read This Book By **neurosurgeon and CNN chief medical correspondent Sanjay Gupta**

" Keep Sharp: Build a Better Brain at Any Age"

Link: https://www.amazon.com/Keep-Sharp-Build-Better-Brain-ebook/dp/B081ZWJ2S8